I0413967

Essential Oils

30 Essential Oil Blends For Aromatherapy Roll-ons

Table of content

Introduction

Your morning went well. You got the kids up and to school on time, dinner is in the slow cooker, waiting for you to get home, and you got all of the morning's assignments done. Lunch time was great, and now you are headed back to work.

And that's when it strikes.

A headache out of the south field, that you weren't ready for, let alone expecting. This is worse than anything you thought you would have to deal with today, and you are out of your Tylenol. If only you were at home so you could toss some peppermint in your diffuser and sit next to the warm fumes as your headache clears.

Or perhaps you are sitting at the office, waiting for your turn in the interview room. You know you are prepared, you have done the prep work, the qualifications, and you wore what you knew would make you stand out from the rest of the crowd, but you feel nervous. If only there was a way to suddenly feel calm and relaxed... but you know you won't be able to slip into the tub until this is all over and done with.

Do these situations sound familiar? Do you ever feel the need to relax, relieve tension, or get away from the pain, but you can't because you are in the middle of your day? If anything like this has ever happened to you, then you know how good it is to have essential oils at your fingertips.

With essential oil roll-ons, you have just what you need right then and there. Completely customized to your own particular need, yet small and discreet so you can use it whenever you want, or whenever you need. This book is going to give you the recipes you need to face anything that comes your way, no matter what it may be.

Headaches, stress, aches and pains that like to creep up on you at the worst times... all of these are going to go away when you have the relief you need right at your fingertips.

So what are you waiting for? Are you tired of the drag you face to get through your day? Now, you can say goodbye to that stress and hello to the easiest essentials ever.

Chapter 1 – Getting Started: Aromatherapy Roll-Ons

As you already know, essential oils have been around for centuries. They are used for a variety of ailments (pretty much any illness that is known to man) and they are limitless.

Now, for a first time user, you may be wondering what the big deal is about the oils.

- Why are they so prevalent?

- Why are they controversial?

- Where do they come from?

- What is the best way to use them?

All of these questions are very common in the essential oil circle, and with good reason. For starters, they are so prevalent because essential oils come from plants. Nearly every essential oil is named for the plant it came from, and in order to get more oils, all you need is more of these plants.

Oils come from all kinds of plants from all over the world, and they are bountiful.

But why are they controversial?

There are those that claim you need to use the lab produced medication in order to feel right, but as soon as you try out any of these oils, you are going to see that isn't the case. Sure, Tylenol or aspirin may do a great job of getting rid of a headache, but why do you need to go to the store to get either one of those when you have plenty of peppermint or chamomile on hand?

As a general rule of thumb, the closer you can get to nature, the better. We are designed to live in this world, and to use the things in this world to heal ourselves and make our lives easier. Nature itself holds a plethora of ways for us to do this, all we need to do is reach out and take it.

If we are responsible, and use the oils properly, we are going to get the good things they have to offer and none of the risks.

What are the risks?

Some oils are dangerous to apply directly to your skin in their pure form. These are very intense oils, and they need to be treated accordingly, which is why you will see in each of the recipes I have down below, I have included the carrier oil in the list.

The reason I said you can choose the carrier oil is because you are free to make your own decision here. Popular carrier oils include:

- Coconut oil

- Olive oil

- Grapeseed oil

- Any specifically named carrier oil (can be a variety of oils)

These oils are entirely safe to apply to your skin, and they dilute the essential oils enough to prevent them from causing any ill side effects by applying them directly to your skin. Always always always use a carrier oil, no matter what you think you can withstand.

For each of the recipes below, I have the amount of drops listed for each, and the carrier oil of your choice. For the standard recipes, I recommend you use 1 tablespoon carrier oil per recipe. If you double the recipe, double the carrier.

For each of the recipes, make them in their entirety, including the carrier oil, then place them in the rollers. This will ensure that each of the oils has been diluted down to a safe level for you to use directly on your skin, no matter how much you put in the roller.

Is rolling the oils onto my skin the best way to use them?

Essential oils are used through the method of aromatherapy. This means you don't have to ingest them for them to work, but rather, smelling them is what makes them work for you. You can do this in two ways.

The most common way to use essential oils is through a diffuser, but they aren't always the most practical thing to have around you in your busy day. The same goes for the warmers, burners, and the reeds.

When you put them in a roller, you are able to apply them to your skin, where some of the oils are going to be absorbed, and where you are going to be able to enjoy the delicious aroma they put forth. This is going to work out double, as you get the have the intense concentration of the oil along with the milder aromatherapy.

How do I get these rollers, and how do I get the oil inside?

Thankfully, since the practice of the use of oils is gaining more popularity these days, you aren't going to have an issue finding these rollers. They are found in a variety of health food stores, hobby stores, or online. You can find a beautiful selection of them on Amazon, including different sizes for your specific needs.

To fill the rollers, all you need to do is use an eye dropper, a toothpick, or a fine funnel to line up the oil with the jar, and pour the oil in slowly. The ball is going to be attached to a screw cap on the jar, and to get it off you only need to unscrew it and you are ready to pour it in!

Fill the bottles to the top, there is no need to leave any space at the top for any reason. Of course, you are going to find a set of instructions with each of the bottles you buy, so there's no need to stress.

That's all you need to know when it comes to the rollers, because it really is as simple as that. They are incredibly user friendly, so all you really need to focus on is the oils you want for your recipes, and the blends themselves. In no time at all you are going to be hooked on these rollers, and you are going to have an answer for any illness or bit of stress that comes your way.

In fact, you are going to discover just how easy it is to make your own oils, and you can soon mix them to suit your own needs and wants. Have fun with this, and see what oils work best for you, and how you like them.

Now, let's get into the recipes.

Chapter 2 – The Good Mooditudes

Let's face it, we can all use that little pick-me-up in the afternoon from time to time. Or in the morning, or really, any time of the day. No matter where you are, what you are doing, or what time of day it is, these are the oils to bring your mood up and keep it there.

You can be glad that you feel better, happy that you didn't have to take any kind of medication, and breeze through your afternoon knowing you will be able to sleep well without pumping yourself full of the caffeine you are normally tempted to reach for.

These oils are the perfect go to for any of your low moods. Use them once, and you can expect to be up and running again in no time!

Afternoon Pick Me Up

What you will need:

5 drops chamomile

5 drops frankincense

5 drops bergamot

Carrier oil of your choice

Carrier oil of your choice

Directions:

Blend the oils with your carrier oil, and mix well. Transfer into your roll-on bottle(s) and screw on the lid tightly.

When you are ready to use, spread across your forehead, from your ears down the back of your jawline, or on your wrists.

If you are needing a larger dose, you can roll the oils onto all three places.

The Sonic Tonic

What you will need:

10 drops wild orange

5 drops lemongrass

3 drops roman chamomile

Carrier oil of your choice

Directions:

Blend the oils with your carrier oil, and mix well. Transfer into your roll-on bottle(s) and screw on the lid tightly.

When you are ready to use, spread across your forehead, from your ears down the back of your jawline, or on your wrists.

If you are needing a larger dose, you can roll the oils onto all three places.

The Happy Days Deluxe

What you will need:

10 drops sandalwood

5 drops bergamot

5 drops vetiver

Carrier oil of your choice

Directions:

Blend the oils with your carrier oil, and mix well. Transfer into your roll-on bottle(s) and screw on the lid tightly.

When you are ready to use, spread across your forehead, from your ears down the back of your jawline, or on your wrists.

If you are needing a larger dose, you can roll the oils onto all three places.

Every Day Like Christmas

What you will need:

5 drops peppermint

6 drops patchouli

6 drops neroli

4 drops ginger

Carrier oil of your choice

Directions:

Blend the oils with your carrier oil, and mix well. Transfer into your roll-on bottle(s) and screw on the lid tightly.

When you are ready to use, spread across your forehead, from your ears down the back of your jawline, or on your wrists.

If you are needing a larger dose, you can roll the oils onto all three places.

The Laughing Stock Tonic

What you will need:

10 drops lavender

5 drops wild orange

5 drops ylang ylang

5 drops rosemary

Carrier oil of your choice

Directions:

Blend the oils with your carrier oil, and mix well. Transfer into your roll-on bottle(s) and screw on the lid tightly.

When you are ready to use, spread across your forehead, from your ears down the back of your jawline, or on your wrists.

If you are needing a larger dose, you can roll the oils onto all three places.

Chapter 3 – Essential Essences

It can be hard to look your best in the fast paced world that you live in. It's hard enough to find a few minutes to relax, let alone the time to get in the spa, massages, or any other treatment you need to pamper yourself.

So what can you do? Let it all go to waste? No! With these oil blends on hand, you have what you need right at your fingertips to look your youthful best. Whether you want to get rid of a few wrinkles that seem to think they are welcome, want to bring back that strong shine your hair used to have, or make those brittle nails as tough as actual nails... these are the blends for you.

Spread them on, work them in, and do what you need to do to make your youthful you come back! You are going to fall in love with the results, so don't hesitate to give it your all.

The Wrinkle Eraser

What you will need:

8 drops myrrh

8 drops sandalwood

5 drops carrot seed

Carrier oil of your choice

Directions:

Blend the oils with your carrier oil, and mix well. Transfer into your roll-on bottle(s) and screw on the lid tightly.

When you are ready to use, spread across your forehead, or across your cheeks. Use your fingers to work it in around your eyes, but only the skin that is near your eyes, not the soft skin that is directly under them.

When you use this oil blend frequently, you will see a massive improvement, but you must be careful not to get any in your eyes.

The Bright Eyes – Use as directed, do not put in eyes!

What you will need:

10 drops frankincense

5 drops helichrysum

10 drops cypress

Carrier oil of your choice

Directions:

Blend the oils with your carrier oil, and mix well. Transfer into your roll-on bottle(s) and screw on the lid tightly.

When you are ready to use, spread across your forehead, from your ears down the back of your jawline, or on your wrists.

If you are needing a larger dose, you can roll the oils onto all three places.

The Tougher Than Nails Blend

What you will need:

10 drops jojoba

10 drops lemon

10 drops lavender

Carrier oil of your choice

Directions:

Blend the oils with your carrier oil, and mix well. Transfer into your roll-on bottle(s) and screw on the lid tightly.

When you are ready to use, spread across your palm, and work over your fingers, massaging the oil in over your nails. If you would like more concentrated application, roll the oil directly on your nails.

Use daily.

Sleek And Shiny Mane Blend

What you will need:

10 drops cedarwood oil

5 drops clary sage oil

5 drops vetiver

5 drops ylang ylang

Carrier oil of your choice

Directions:

Blend the oils with your carrier oil, and mix well. Transfer into your roll-on bottle(s) and screw on the lid tightly.

When you are ready to use, spread a generous amount on the palm of your hand, and work through your hair. Repeat as many times as you would like, and rinse well.

You may also spread some on your hand, then lather with your shampoo before you wash your hair. Rinse well.

The Breath Of Fresh Air

What you will need:

8 drops eucalyptus

8 drops peppermint

5 drops lavender

Carrier oil of your choice

Directions:

Blend the oils with your carrier oil, and mix well. Transfer into your roll-on bottle(s) and screw on the lid tightly.

When you are ready to use, spread across your forehead, from your ears down the back of your jawline, or on your wrists.

If you are needing a larger dose, you can roll the oils onto all three places.

Chapter 4 – For The Young Or Young At Heart

It really doesn't matter if you are young at heart, or if you are doing this for your little ones who are, these are the blends that you absolutely need to have on hand. They are perfect to help get rid of those hormonal things that happen to the young'uns, and they are that little boost of confidence and happiness they need from time to time.

Of course, we all need that little boost every now and then, and there are those little annoyances that like to pop up that we like to get rid of. These oils don't care how old you are, they are going to help you get what you want no matter what.

Keep each of these blends on hand at all times, and say goodbye to those little difficulties that like to crop up every now and then.

The Acne Blaster

What you will need:

8 drops tea tree oil

8 drops clary sage

5 drops juniper

Carrier oil of your choice

Directions:

Blend the oils with your carrier oil, and mix well. Transfer into your roll-on bottle(s) and screw on the lid tightly.

When you are ready to use, spread across your forehead, from your ears down the back of your jawline, or on your wrists.

If you are needing a larger dose, you can roll the oils onto all three places.

The Goodnight Moonbeam

What you will need:

6 drops lavender

4 drops chamomile

1 drop eucalyptus

Carrier oil of your choice

Directions:

Blend the oils with your carrier oil, and mix well. Transfer into your roll-on bottle(s) and screw on the lid tightly.

When you are ready to use, spread across your forehead, from your ears down the back of your jawline, or on your wrists.

If you are needing a larger dose, you can roll the oils onto all three places.

The Tummy Tickler

What you will need:

10 drops peppermint

5 drops lemon

5 drops ginger essential oil

Carrier oil of your choice

Directions:

Blend the oils with your carrier oil, and mix well. Transfer into your roll-on bottle(s) and screw on the lid tightly.

When you are ready to use, spread across your forehead, from your ears down the back of your jawline, or on your wrists.

If you are needing a larger dose, you can roll the oils onto all three places.

The Booboo Bandaid

What you will need:

12 drops myrrh

5 drops tea tree

3 drops orange

Carrier oil of your choice

Directions:

Blend the oils with your carrier oil, and mix well. Transfer into your roll-on bottle(s) and screw on the lid tightly.

When you are ready to use, spread across your forehead, from your ears down the back of your jawline, or on your wrists.

If you are needing a larger dose, you can roll the oils onto all three places.

A Hug From Mom

What you will need:

5 drops lavender

5 drops marjoram

5 drops ylang ylang

5 drops palmarosa

5 drops rose

Carrier oil of your choice

Directions:

Blend the oils with your carrier oil, and mix well. Transfer into your roll-on bottle(s) and screw on the lid tightly.

When you are ready to use, spread across your forehead, from your ears down the back of your jawline, or on your wrists.

If you are needing a larger dose, you can roll the oils onto all three places.

Chapter 5 – For The Aches And Pains

Whether you are into sports, work with your hands a lot, or are just experiencing the natural flow of life, you know what it is like to have those little aches and pains come into play every now and then. While they had you running for some aspirin before, these are going to fade away now that you have your blends on hand.

You know you would like to have that youthful vigor back, and when you erase those aches and pains it's right there, as though it hadn't ever disappeared. These oils are going to help your cramps and aches go away, as well as help those joints move as they once did. You're going to feel like your old self again in no time at all!

Get ready for a new kind of freedom... the freedom to move!

The Headache Hustler

What you will need:

10 drops sweet marjoram

3 drops peppermint

5 drops rosemary

Carrier oil of your choice

Directions:

Blend the oils with your carrier oil, and mix well. Transfer into your roll-on bottle(s) and screw on the lid tightly.

When you are ready to use, spread across your forehead, from your ears down the back of your jawline, or on your wrists.

If you are needing a larger dose, you can roll the oils onto all three places.

The Incredible Joint Juice

What you will need:

5 drops peppermint

10 drops juniper

10 drops yarrow

Carrier oil of your choice

Directions:

Blend the oils with your carrier oil, and mix well. Transfer into your roll-on bottle(s) and screw on the lid tightly.

When you are ready to use, spread across your forehead, from your ears down the back of your jawline, or on your wrists.

If you are needing a larger dose, you can roll the oils onto all three places.

The Hop Scotch (for those PMSing days)

What you will need:

10 drops wintergreen

10 drops clary sage

5 drops yarrow

Carrier oil of your choice

Directions:

Blend the oils with your carrier oil, and mix well. Transfer into your roll-on bottle(s) and screw on the lid tightly.

When you are ready to use, spread across your forehead, from your ears down the back of your jawline, or on your wrists.

If you are needing a larger dose, you can roll the oils onto all three places.

The Ache-Away

What you will need:

10 drops helichrysum

5 drops chamomile

5 drops vetiver

Carrier oil of your choice

Directions:

Blend the oils with your carrier oil, and mix well. Transfer into your roll-on bottle(s) and screw on the lid tightly.

When you are ready to use, spread across your forehead, from your ears down the back of your jawline, or on your wrists.

If you are needing a larger dose, you can roll the oils onto all three places.

Field of Dreams

What you will need:

5 drops lavender

5 drops chamomile

5 drops frankincense

5 drops ginger

Carrier oil of your choice

Directions:

Blend the oils with your carrier oil, and mix well. Transfer into your roll-on bottle(s) and screw on the lid tightly.

When you are ready to use, spread across your forehead, from your ears down the back of your jawline, or on your wrists.

If you are needing a larger dose, you can roll the oils onto all three places.

Chapter 6 – Healthy Blasts

It seems that health and fitness are all over the place these days, and it is a small wonder why. Nothing is more important than your health, and nothing is more valuable than getting it back or keeping it at its prime.

But, with busy days and hardly any time for yourself, let alone for enough sleep, your health is one of the first things to go downhill when you start to get rundown. That is why these blends are so essential to have with you at all times.

Whether you need that little boost to keep your health at its prime, or if you want that little boost to scare off any cold or flu that is trying to creep its way in, these are the blends for you.

The amount of benefits you are going to get from these blends is more than I can list, so give them a try and see the good things come rolling in. Use them for the ailment they are intended for, and you are going to see your health increase in other areas as well.

This is a total win for you and anyone around you. Think of it as your little healing potion in a bottle.

The Cold and Flu Buster

What you will need:

5 drops tea tree

10 drops pine

5 drops thyme

5 drops thieves

Carrier oil of your choice

Directions:

Blend the oils with your carrier oil, and mix well. Transfer into your roll-on bottle(s) and screw on the lid tightly.

When you are ready to use, spread across your forehead, from your ears down the back of your jawline, or on your wrists.

If you are needing a larger dose, you can roll the oils onto all three places.

The Infection Fighter

What you will need:

10 drops geranium

10 drops cinnamon bark

5 drops lemongrass

2 drops rosemary

Carrier oil of your choice

Directions:

Blend the oils with your carrier oil, and mix well. Transfer into your roll-on bottle(s) and screw on the lid tightly.

When you are ready to use, spread across your forehead, from your ears down the back of your jawline, or on your wrists.

If you are needing a larger dose, you can roll the oils onto all three places.

The Superman Blend

What you will need:

5 drops garlic

10 drops ginger

10 drops eucalyptus

5 drops tea tree

Carrier oil of your choice

Directions:

Blend the oils with your carrier oil, and mix well. Transfer into your roll-on bottle(s) and screw on the lid tightly.

When you are ready to use, spread across your forehead, from your ears down the back of your jawline, or on your wrists.

If you are needing a larger dose, you can roll the oils onto all three places.

The Immunity Guard

What you will need:

10 drops thieves

10 drops valor

5 drops lavender

Carrier oil of your choice

Directions:

Blend the oils with your carrier oil, and mix well. Transfer into your roll-on bottle(s) and screw on the lid tightly.

When you are ready to use, spread across your forehead, from your ears down the back of your jawline, or on your wrists.

If you are needing a larger dose, you can roll the oils onto all three places.

The Day Saver

What you will need:

10 drops peppermint

5 drops bergamot

5 drops myrrh

4 drops goldenseal

4 drops lemongrass

Carrier oil of your choice

Directions:

Blend the oils with your carrier oil, and mix well. Transfer into your roll-on bottle(s) and screw on the lid tightly.

When you are ready to use, spread across your forehead, from your ears down the back of your jawline, or on your wrists.

If you are needing a larger dose, you can roll the oils onto all three places.

Conclusion

There you have it, everything you need to know about the essential roll-ons you need for your purse, pocket, backpack, or anywhere else you want. With the ease of these aromatherapy roll-ons, you don't have to stress about where your oils are, how you are going to blend them, or if they are going to leak in your car. With these roll-ons, you have all the help and relief you need in the most convenient way possible.

Say hello to a stress free day when you pack these into your purse. It doesn't matter what you are going to do with your day, if you have these by your side, you are going to be ready to face all kinds of challenges that head your way.

Shake off the stress, the illness, and the aches with the flick of your wrist, and when you want that extra little boost, spread some on your chest or neck as well. There's no limit to the ways essentials are going to better your life, and you are going to fall in love with the results.

Your spouse, your children, and even your friends can be helped when you have just a few drops of these oils on hand, and when you are able to step that up even further by bringing an entire collection with you, there is nothing that can stop you from having a good day.

So toss out all of your concern and your stress, and get ready for the best carry-on you can imagine. This book is going to be your guide when it comes to the essentials, so don't be afraid to jump right on in and give it all you got.

Your health is going to be better off in every aspect, and you won't ever want to be caught without any of these blends on hand again.

www.ingramcontent.com/pod-product-compliance
Lightning Source LLC
Chambersburg PA
CBHW071153280526
45787CB00003B/1501